ONE MEAL A DAY COOKBOOK

Delicious And Nutritious OMAD Recipes: Simple Meals For Breakfast, Lunch, Dinner, And Desserts

Charlotte Harry

Table of Contents

CHAPTER ONE

INTRODUCTION TO ONE MEAL A DAY (OMAD)

What Is Omad?

One Meal a Day (OMAD) is a form of intermittent fasting that has gained popularity for its simplicity and potential health benefits. As the name suggests, OMAD involves consuming all of one's daily caloric intake within a single meal, typically within a designated one-hour eating window. The remainder of the day is spent fasting, during which no food is consumed. However, beverages such as water, tea, and black coffee are generally permitted, making the fasting period more manageable.

This eating pattern appeals to many due to its straightforward nature. By limiting food consumption to just one meal, individuals can simplify their daily routines. OMAD can be particularly advantageous for those who struggle to find the time or energy to prepare and eat multiple meals throughout the day. It allows for flexibility in meal timing, enabling individuals to choose the most convenient meal, whether that be breakfast, lunch, or dinner.

While OMAD may seem restrictive, it encourages people to focus on the quality of their meals. The key to successful OMAD practice is ensuring that the single meal consumed meets one's nutritional needs, providing adequate protein, healthy fats, and carbohydrates, as well as vitamins and minerals. This approach promotes mindfulness around food choices, encouraging individuals to prioritize nutrient-dense foods over processed options.

Moreover, OMAD may offer several health benefits. Some proponents suggest that this eating pattern can lead to weight loss, as it often results in a reduction in overall calorie intake. The fasting period may also enhance metabolic health, improve insulin sensitivity, and support cellular repair processes. Additionally, many people report increased mental clarity and focus during the fasting hours, attributing it to the absence of post-meal drowsiness.

It's important to note that OMAD may not be suitable for everyone. Individuals with certain health conditions, those who are pregnant or breastfeeding, or those with a history of disordered eating should consult a healthcare professional before adopting this approach. Listening to one's body is crucial, as some may find fasting challenging or may not feel satiated with just one meal.

Benefits Of Omad

The One Meal a Day (OMAD) approach to eating has gained popularity for its potential health benefits, particularly regarding weight management and metabolic health. One of the most significant advantages of OMAD is its efficacy in promoting weight loss. By limiting the eating window to just one meal per day, individuals often experience a natural reduction in calorie intake. This restricted eating pattern can lead to significant weight loss, as many find it easier to consume fewer calories within a shorter time frame. Additionally, the fasting periods associated with OMAD can stimulate metabolic processes that enhance fat burning, making it a viable option for those looking to shed extra pounds.

Beyond weight loss, OMAD is linked to several improvements in metabolic health. Research indicates that intermittent fasting, including OMAD, can boost insulin sensitivity, a crucial factor in preventing type 2 diabetes. Improved insulin sensitivity allows the body to process glucose more effectively, reducing the risk of spikes in blood sugar levels. Furthermore, OMAD may help reduce inflammation, a contributor to numerous chronic health issues, thereby promoting overall well-being. The cellular repair processes activated during fasting periods can lead to better health outcomes, including enhanced longevity.

Heart health is another area where OMAD shows promise. Studies suggest that regular fasting can lower cholesterol levels and reduce blood pressure, both of which are vital for cardiovascular health. By adopting OMAD, individuals may reduce their risk of heart disease and related complications, leading to a healthier lifestyle overall.

In addition to its physical benefits, OMAD offers practical advantages. With only one meal to prepare each day, individuals can save significant time in the kitchen. This simplicity can make meal planning more straightforward, allowing for easier grocery shopping and meal prep. For many, this streamlined approach to eating is appealing, especially for those with busy schedules.

Moreover, numerous OMAD practitioners report enhanced mental clarity and focus during fasting periods. This boost in cognitive function may be attributed to the body's shift in energy use from glucose to fat, which can result in a more stable energy supply. As the body becomes accustomed to this alternative energy source, many experience improved concentration and productivity throughout the day.

Getting Started With Omad

Getting started with OMAD (One Meal a Day) journey can be both exciting and transformative. This method of intermittent fasting focuses on consuming all your daily calories in a single meal, allowing for a prolonged fasting period that can benefit various aspects of health, including weight loss, improved metabolism, and enhanced mental clarity.

To begin, the first step is to select a meal that aligns with your personal schedule and lifestyle. Whether you choose lunch or dinner depends on when you typically experience the most hunger or when you have the time to fully enjoy and prepare your meal. Understanding your body's rhythms is crucial, as it will set you up for success in adhering to the OMAD routine.

A gradual approach to shifting your eating habits is highly recommended. If you currently have three meals a day, consider starting by reducing your eating window to two meals before transitioning to one. This incremental adjustment can help minimize feelings of hunger and discomfort as your body adapts to a new eating pattern. Pay attention to your hunger cues and allow your body the time it needs to adjust.

When it comes to preparing your one meal, it's essential to create a balanced plate. Focus on incorporating a variety of nutrients by including a source of protein—such as chicken, fish, beans, or tofu—along with healthy fats like avocados, olive oil, or nuts. Whole grains can provide essential carbohydrates, while a generous serving of vegetables will ensure you're meeting your fiber needs and receiving vital vitamins and minerals.

Another important aspect of the OMAD lifestyle is hydration. Staying well-hydrated throughout the day is crucial, as it not only supports overall health but can also help manage hunger pangs. Drinking water, herbal teas, or other non-caloric beverages can aid in maintaining a feeling of fullness, making it easier to adhere to your fasting period.

As you start with OMAD, listen to your body and adjust as needed. Each individual's experience with intermittent fasting can vary, so be flexible and responsive to how you feel. Remember that consistency is key, and over time, OMAD can become a sustainable part of your lifestyle, bringing with it a host of potential health benefits. Enjoy the journey, and savor the experience of creating and relishing your one daily meal!

Tips For Success

One Meal a Day (OMAD) can be an effective approach to intermittent fasting, but like any dietary strategy, it requires careful consideration and planning. Here are some essential tips to help you succeed with OMAD.

1. Listen to Your Body:

The foundation of any successful diet is tuning into your body's signals. During the fasting and eating periods, pay close attention to how you feel. If you experience excessive fatigue, persistent hunger, or discomfort, it might be a sign to reassess your approach. Every individual's body responds differently to fasting, so be willing to make adjustments that best suit your needs.

2. Plan Your Meals:

Meal planning is crucial when practicing OMAD. Take the time to decide what you will eat during your designated meal time. Planning helps ensure that your meal is balanced, nutritious, and satisfying, which can prevent the urge to indulge in unhealthy options. By preparing your meal in advance, you can include a variety of food groups—proteins, healthy fats, and plenty of vegetables—to meet your nutritional needs and keep you feeling full.

3. Stay Consistent:

Consistency is key in establishing any new routine. While it's important to be flexible, try to adhere to your chosen eating window regularly. This consistency helps your body adapt to the OMAD schedule, optimizing the benefits you experience over time. Establishing a routine can also make it easier to plan your meals and manage hunger.

4. Stay Active:

Incorporating regular physical activity into your daily routine can enhance the benefits of OMAD. Exercise not only helps in managing hunger but also boosts overall health and well-being. Whether it's a brisk walk, strength training, or yoga, finding an activity you enjoy can make staying active easier and more enjoyable. Aim for a balance between exercise and rest to ensure your body can recover and thrive.

5. Seek Support:

Embarking on an OMAD journey can be more manageable and enjoyable with support. Consider joining a community or finding a buddy who shares your interest in OMAD. Sharing experiences, recipes, and tips can keep you motivated and provide accountability. Whether online or in-person, support networks can make a significant difference in your success and adherence to the OMAD lifestyle.

CHAPTER TWO

PLANNING YOUR OMAD MEALS

Understanding Nutritional Needs

When planning your One Meal A Day (OMAD) meals, understanding your nutritional needs is paramount. Every individual's body has unique requirements, so it's essential to grasp what nutrients you need to stay healthy and energized. These nutrients encompass macronutrients such as carbohydrates, proteins, and fats, alongside micronutrients like vitamins and minerals.

Carbohydrates, proteins, and fats play critical roles in maintaining bodily functions. Carbohydrates are the body's primary energy source, fueling daily activities and ensuring that both the brain and muscles perform optimally. Simple carbohydrates, like those found in fruits and dairy, provide quick energy, while complex carbohydrates from whole grains and vegetables offer sustained energy release throughout the day.

Proteins are the building blocks of the body, crucial for muscle repair and growth, tissue maintenance, and the production of enzymes and hormones. High-quality protein sources include lean meats, poultry, fish, eggs, dairy products, legumes, and nuts. Ensuring adequate protein intake is particularly important in an OMAD diet to support muscle health and recovery, especially if you engage in regular physical activity.

Fats, often misunderstood, are essential for numerous bodily functions. They aid in cell structure, hormone production, and nutrient absorption. Healthy fats, such as those from avocados, nuts, seeds, and olive oil, should be prioritized. Omega-3 fatty acids, found in fatty fish like salmon and flaxseeds, are particularly beneficial for heart health and inflammation reduction.

Micronutrients, while needed in smaller quantities, are equally vital. Vitamins such as A, B, C, D, E, and K, and minerals like calcium, magnesium, potassium, and iron, support a range of bodily functions. For instance, vitamin A is essential for vision and immune function, B vitamins play a role in energy metabolism, vitamin C is crucial for tissue repair and immune support, and vitamin D facilitates calcium absorption for bone health. Minerals like calcium and magnesium are necessary for bone and muscle health, while potassium regulates fluid balance and iron is vital for oxygen transport in the blood.

To accurately determine your specific nutritional needs, consulting with a nutritionist can be highly beneficial. They can provide personalized guidance based on factors such as age, gender, weight, activity level, and health goals. Alternatively, various online calculators can offer a good baseline, factoring in these elements to help you understand your daily requirements.

Meal Prep And Planning

Understanding your nutritional needs is the first step towards successful meal prep and planning, especially when following the One Meal a Day (OMAD) intermittent fasting approach. Once you've identified your dietary requirements, planning and preparing your meals in advance becomes crucial. Not only does this practice save time, but it also ensures that you adhere to your dietary goals without deviation.

Begin by establishing a weekly menu. This involves selecting a variety of dishes that you enjoy and that align with your nutritional needs. Including diverse foods is essential to prevent monotony and to guarantee a comprehensive intake of nutrients. Variety in your diet helps to keep your meals exciting and nutritionally balanced, contributing to overall better adherence to your dietary plan.

Once your menu is set, the next step is to create a detailed grocery list. A well-thought-out list serves multiple purposes: it prevents impulsive buying, ensures that you purchase only what is necessary, and helps you to stay within your budget. Moreover, having a complete list means you won't find yourself missing key ingredients when it's time to prepare your meals.

Dedicate a specific time each week to meal prep. Many people find that spending a few hours on a Sunday afternoon works well, but you can choose any day that fits your schedule. During this time, focus on prepping ingredients and even cooking some components of your meals. For example, you can chop vegetables, cook grains such as rice or quinoa, and prepare proteins like chicken, fish, or tofu. These prepped ingredients can then be stored in the refrigerator or freezer, ready to be assembled into meals throughout the week.

Meal prepping offers numerous benefits. Firstly, it reduces the daily burden of cooking, making it easier to stick to your OMAD regimen. With healthy, pre-prepared options available, you are less likely to resort to unhealthy, quick fixes when hunger strikes. Additionally, meal prep encourages portion control and mindful eating, both of which are crucial for maintaining your health and achieving your dietary goals.

To further enhance your meal prep routine, consider investing in quality storage containers. These containers keep your prepped food fresh and make it easy to portion out your meals. Labeling containers with the contents and the date prepared can also be helpful for keeping track of your food.

Grocery shopping is an essential part of meal planning, especially for those following the One Meal a Day (OMAD) diet. To make the most out of your shopping trips and ensure you're buying the best foods for your OMAD diet, consider these helpful tips:

Make a List and Stick to It

Having a shopping list is crucial for staying focused and avoiding impulse buys that might not align with your dietary goals. Before heading to the store, plan your meals for the week and write down everything you need. This not only saves time but also helps you avoid purchasing unnecessary items. A well-thought-out list ensures you get all the ingredients required for your meals and reduces the chances of buying processed foods or snacks that can derail your diet.

Shop the Perimeter

The outer aisles of grocery stores usually contain fresh produce, meats, dairy, and whole foods, which are more nutritious and less processed than items found in the inner aisles. Fresh fruits and vegetables, lean meats, fish, dairy products, and eggs are often located around the store's perimeter. These foods are the foundation of a healthy OMAD diet as they provide essential nutrients and are minimally processed. Focusing on the perimeter helps you fill your cart with wholesome, nutrient-dense foods.

Choose Whole Foods

Opt for whole, unprocessed foods like fruits, vegetables, lean meats, whole grains, and healthy fats. These foods provide more nutrients and fewer empty calories compared to processed foods. Whole foods are packed with vitamins, minerals, fiber, and other essential nutrients that support overall health and well-being. When you prioritize whole foods, you're more likely to meet your nutritional needs and maintain energy levels throughout the day.

Read Labels

For any packaged foods, read the labels to understand what you're buying. Look for items with fewer ingredients and those that are low in added sugars, unhealthy fats, and artificial additives. Understanding food labels helps you make informed choices and avoid products that contain hidden sugars, trans fats, and other undesirable ingredients. Aim for products with recognizable, whole-food ingredients and minimal additives to ensure you're consuming high-quality foods.

Buy in Bulk

Items like grains, nuts, and seeds can often be bought in bulk, which can be more economical and environmentally friendly. Buying in bulk allows you to purchase larger quantities at a lower cost per unit, reducing packaging waste and saving money in the long run. Stocking up on bulk items ensures you always have healthy staples on hand, making it easier to prepare nutritious meals without frequent trips to the store.

Balancing Macronutrients

Balancing macronutrients is essential in an OMAD (One Meal A Day) diet because you need to get all your essential nutrients in a single meal. Achieving this balance ensures that your body receives the necessary fuel for energy, muscle repair, and overall health, despite the limited eating window. Here's how you can effectively balance your macronutrients in an OMAD diet:

Carbohydrates: Carbohydrates should constitute about 40-50% of your meal. Focus on complex carbohydrates such as whole grains, fruits, and vegetables. These provide sustained energy and are rich in fiber, which is important for digestive health and helps you feel full longer. Examples of complex carbohydrates include quinoa, brown rice, sweet potatoes, and a variety of fruits and vegetables like berries, apples, broccoli, and spinach. These foods not only provide energy but also supply essential vitamins and minerals that support overall well-being.

Proteins: Proteins should account for about 25-30% of your meal. Lean sources of protein such as chicken, fish, legumes, and tofu are ideal choices. Protein is vital for muscle repair and maintenance, especially if you engage in regular physical activity. It also plays a crucial role in the production of enzymes and hormones, supporting various bodily functions. Incorporating a variety of protein sources ensures you get a range of amino acids, which are the building blocks of protein. For example, combining beans with rice provides a complete protein profile, making it an excellent choice for vegetarians and vegans.

Fats: Healthy fats should make up about 20-30% of your meal. These fats are important for cell function, hormone production, and the absorption of fat-soluble vitamins (A, D, E, and K). Good sources of healthy fats include avocados, nuts, seeds, and olive oil. Incorporating these fats into your diet helps maintain healthy skin, supports brain health, and provides a concentrated source of energy. For instance, adding a handful of almonds or a tablespoon of chia seeds to your meal can boost your intake of omega-3 fatty acids, which are beneficial for heart health.

CHAPTER THREE

BREAKFAST-INSPIRED OMAD RECIPES

Savory Breakfast Bowls

Savory breakfast bowls are a versatile and nutritious way to start your day, combining a variety of ingredients to create a balanced and satisfying meal. These bowls typically include a base, such as grains or greens, topped with a mix of proteins, vegetables, and healthy fats. Here's how to create some delicious savory breakfast bowls:

1. Grain-Based Bowls: A popular choice for breakfast bowls is using grains like quinoa, brown rice, or oatmeal. These grains provide a hearty base and are rich in fiber, which helps you feel full longer. To assemble a grain-based bowl, start with a generous scoop of your chosen grain. Top it

with a variety of ingredients such as sautéed spinach, roasted vegetables, and avocado slices. A poached egg adds protein and creaminess to the bowl. To enhance the flavors even more, consider adding a sprinkle of cheese, such as feta or Parmesan, or a drizzle of olive oil. This combination not only tastes great but also provides a range of nutrients to fuel your day.

2. Green-Based Bowls: For those who prefer a lighter base, leafy greens like kale, spinach, or arugula are excellent options. These greens are low in calories but high in essential nutrients, making them a perfect foundation for a nutritious breakfast bowl. Begin with a bed of fresh greens and top it with ingredients like grilled chicken, chickpeas, cherry tomatoes, and a soft-

boiled egg. These toppings add protein, fiber, and a variety of vitamins and minerals to your meal. To bring all the flavors together, a simple vinaigrette made with olive oil, lemon juice, and a touch of Dijon mustard can be drizzled over the top. This green-based bowl is both refreshing and satisfying.

3. Protein-Rich Toppings: Adding protein-rich toppings to your breakfast bowl can make it more filling and help sustain your energy levels throughout the morning. Proteins such as bacon, smoked salmon, or tofu are great options. Bacon provides a savory crunch, smoked salmon offers a rich, smoky flavor, and tofu is a versatile plant-based protein that can be seasoned to your liking. Combine these proteins with your favorite vegetables, such as bell

peppers, mushrooms, or zucchini. A tasty sauce or dressing, like a tahini drizzle or a yogurt-based sauce, can tie all the elements together, creating a delicious and balanced meal.

Protein-Packed Smoothies

Smoothies are a quick and easy way to consume a lot of nutrients in one go. By focusing on protein-packed ingredients, you can create a smoothie that not only tastes good but also keeps you full for hours. Here's how to craft the perfect protein-packed smoothie.

Base Ingredients

Start with a liquid base such as almond milk, coconut water, or Greek yogurt. Almond milk and coconut water are excellent choices if you're looking for a dairy-free option. Almond milk provides a creamy texture and is rich in calcium, while coconut water offers a refreshing taste and is packed with electrolytes, perfect for hydration. Greek yogurt, on the other hand, adds a thicker consistency and is a fantastic source of probiotics, which are beneficial for your digestive health. These base ingredients not only give your smoothie a smooth texture but also contribute essential nutrients.

Protein Boosters

To make your smoothie protein-rich, consider adding ingredients like protein powder, nut butters, or seeds such as chia or flax. Protein powder is a convenient way to significantly increase the protein content of your smoothie, with various flavors available to suit your taste. Nut butters like almond or peanut butter add both protein and healthy fats, enhancing the smoothie's creaminess and keeping you satiated for longer periods. Seeds such as chia and flax are small but mighty, offering a boost of protein, fiber, and omega-3 fatty acids, which are great for heart health.

Fruits and Vegetables

Adding fruits like berries, bananas, and mangoes can give your smoothie a sweet flavor while providing essential vitamins and antioxidants. Berries, particularly blueberries and strawberries, are loaded with antioxidants and vitamins C and K, which are crucial for immune function and skin health. Bananas add natural sweetness and a creamy texture, along with potassium, which helps in maintaining proper heart and muscle function. Mangoes not only sweeten your smoothie but also provide a rich source of vitamins A and C. Leafy greens like spinach or kale can also be added for an extra nutrient boost without altering the taste significantly. These greens are rich in vitamins A, C, and K, as well as iron and fiber, enhancing the nutritional profile of your smoothie.

Extras

Consider adding extras like oats, cacao nibs, or a spoonful of honey for added flavor and texture. Oats can make your smoothie more filling, providing a good dose of fiber and complex carbohydrates. Cacao nibs add a delightful crunch and are packed with antioxidants and magnesium. A spoonful of honey not only sweetens your smoothie naturally but also offers antibacterial properties and a quick energy boost. These little additions can make your smoothie more interesting and enjoyable.

Omelets And Frittatas

Omelets and frittatas are classic breakfast dishes that offer both deliciousness and versatility, making them ideal for incorporating various ingredients into one satisfying meal. These egg-based creations can be customized to suit different tastes and dietary preferences, and they provide an excellent way to start the day with a nutritious boost.

Omelets

An omelet is a delightful dish made from beaten eggs, quickly cooked with butter or oil in a frying pan. The simplicity of an omelet belies its potential for variety, as it serves as a canvas for numerous fillings. Common additions include cheese, ham, mushrooms, bell peppers, onions, and spinach. The technique for creating a perfect omelet involves cooking the eggs until they are just set and then folding them over the chosen fillings. This method ensures that the omelet is cooked to perfection, with a slightly creamy texture and a flavorful filling.

To make an omelet, start by whisking eggs in a bowl, seasoning with salt and pepper. Heat a small amount of butter or oil in a non-stick frying pan over medium heat. Pour in the eggs, allowing them to spread evenly across the pan. As the eggs begin to set, gently lift the edges with a spatula, letting the uncooked eggs flow underneath. Once the eggs are mostly set but still slightly runny on top, add the desired fillings on one half of the omelet. Carefully fold the other half over the fillings and cook for another minute until the eggs are fully set and the cheese, if used, is melted. Slide the omelet onto a plate and serve immediately for a delicious and satisfying breakfast.

Frittatas

A frittata is a dish similar to an omelet but cooked more slowly and not folded. It usually starts on the stovetop and finishes in the oven, allowing for a different texture and cooking style. Frittatas are excellent for incorporating various ingredients directly into the eggs before cooking. Potatoes, zucchini, cheese, and herbs are popular choices, creating a hearty and flavorful dish.

To make a frittata, preheat the oven to 375°F (190°C). Whisk eggs in a bowl and season with salt and pepper. Heat an oven-safe skillet over medium heat and add a bit of oil or butter. Sauté your chosen ingredients, such as diced potatoes or sliced zucchini, until they are tender. Pour the whisked eggs over the vegetables, stirring gently to combine. Cook on the stovetop until the edges begin to set, then transfer the skillet to the preheated oven. Bake for about 10-15 minutes or until the frittata is fully set and slightly golden on top. Remove from the oven and let it cool slightly before slicing into wedges.

Frittatas are not only delicious but also practical. They are perfect for feeding a crowd and can be made ahead of time, making them ideal for meal prep. They can be served hot, cold, or at room temperature, and they reheat well, ensuring a quick and convenient breakfast or brunch option.

Healthy Pancakes And Waffles

Pancakes and waffles, beloved breakfast staples, can be made healthier by incorporating whole-grain flours and adding nutritious ingredients. With a few simple tweaks, these breakfast favorites can become both indulgent and nutritious, making them a perfect way to start your day.

Whole-Grain Flours

One of the easiest ways to make pancakes and waffles healthier is by using whole-grain flours instead of refined flour. Whole-wheat flour, oat flour, and almond flour are excellent alternatives. These options provide more fiber and nutrients, which not only make your breakfast more filling but also contribute to better overall health. Whole-wheat flour is rich in vitamins and minerals, including iron, calcium, and B vitamins, which are essential for energy and metabolism. Oat flour, made from ground oats, offers a good source of soluble fiber, which can help reduce cholesterol levels. Almond flour, made from finely ground almonds, is packed with protein, healthy fats, and vitamin E, making it a great gluten-free option.

Adding Fruits and Veggies

Incorporating fruits and vegetables into your pancake and waffle batter is another excellent way to boost their nutritional value. Fruits like blueberries, bananas, and grated apples can add natural sweetness and essential vitamins and minerals. Blueberries are high in antioxidants, which help protect your body from damage by free radicals. Bananas are rich in potassium, which is important for heart health and maintaining proper muscle function. Grated apples can add a subtle sweetness and moisture to the batter, along with a dose of vitamin C and fiber. Vegetables such as shredded zucchini or carrots can also be added to the batter without significantly altering the taste. Zucchini is low in calories and high in vitamins A and C, while carrots are a great source of beta-carotene, which your body converts into vitamin A.

Healthy Toppings

The toppings you choose can also make a big difference in the healthiness of your pancakes and waffles. Instead of drowning them in syrup, consider healthier alternatives like fresh fruit, Greek yogurt, nut butter, or a drizzle of honey. Fresh fruit adds natural sweetness and a variety of vitamins and minerals. Greek yogurt provides a good source of protein and probiotics, which are beneficial for gut health. Nut butter, such as almond or peanut butter, adds healthy fats and protein, making your breakfast more satisfying. A drizzle of honey can provide a touch of sweetness while offering antioxidants and antibacterial properties.

CHAPTER FOUR

LUNCH-INSPIRED OMAD RECIPES

Hearty Salads

Salads are a versatile and refreshing option for your OMAD (One Meal A Day) lunch. They can be light yet filling, packed with nutrients and flavors. Hearty salads are more substantial than your average side salad, often including a mix of protein, healthy fats, and a variety of vegetables. Here are some delicious and nourishing hearty salads that will keep you satisfied throughout your fasting period.

Protein-Packed Chicken Caesar Salad

A classic Chicken Caesar Salad is an excellent choice for a hearty OMAD lunch. Start with a bed of crisp romaine lettuce, which provides a satisfying crunch and a base rich in vitamins. Add slices of grilled chicken breast, a lean source of protein that will help keep you full and energized. Toss the lettuce and chicken with a creamy Caesar dressing, which adds a rich and tangy flavor to the salad. Sprinkle on some freshly grated Parmesan cheese for an extra layer of savory goodness. Finally, top with crunchy croutons for texture and additional flavor. This salad is a perfect balance of protein, healthy fats, and carbohydrates, making it a well-rounded meal.

Quinoa and Roasted Veggie Salad

For a vegetarian option, a Quinoa and Roasted Veggie Salad is a fantastic choice. Quinoa is a superfood grain that is high in protein and fiber, making it an excellent base for a hearty salad. Cook the quinoa according to the package instructions and let it cool. Meanwhile, roast a variety of vegetables like bell peppers, zucchini, and cherry tomatoes until they are tender and slightly caramelized. Combine the cooked quinoa with the roasted vegetables and add some crumbled feta cheese, which provides a tangy and creamy element. Dress the salad with a lemon vinaigrette made from fresh lemon juice, olive oil, salt, and pepper. This salad is not only delicious but also packed with nutrients, including vitamins, minerals, and antioxidants.

Tuna Nicoise Salad

A Tuna Nicoise Salad is a French-inspired dish that is both hearty and flavorful. Start with a bed of mixed greens, such as baby spinach, arugula, and lettuce. Add chunks of tuna, which is rich in protein and omega-3 fatty acids. Include hard-boiled eggs for additional protein and healthy fats. Blanch some green beans until they are tender-crisp, and add them to the salad along with boiled potatoes, which provide satisfying carbohydrates. Finish with a handful of olives and cherry tomatoes for a burst of flavor and color. Dress the salad with a mustard vinaigrette made from Dijon mustard, olive oil, red wine vinegar, and a touch of garlic. This salad is a complete meal that combines protein, healthy fats, and a variety of vegetables, ensuring you get a wide range of nutrients in your OMAD meal.

Grain bowls are an excellent lunch option, offering a balanced mix of grains, proteins, and vegetables. They are highly customizable, allowing you to create a meal that suits your taste and dietary needs. Whether you are in the mood for Mediterranean flavors, a Mexican-inspired dish, or an Asian twist, there is a grain bowl for you.

Mediterranean Farro Bowl

Farro is a nutty ancient grain that pairs well with Mediterranean ingredients, making it a delicious and nutritious choice for a grain bowl. To create a Mediterranean Farro Bowl, start with a base of cooked farro. Farro's chewy texture and nutty flavor provide a perfect foundation for the other ingredients. Combine the farro with chickpeas for added protein and fiber. Next, add chopped cucumbers, which bring a refreshing crunch, and juicy tomatoes for a burst of sweetness. Red onion adds a mild, sharp flavor that complements the other ingredients. Top the bowl with crumbled feta cheese, which adds a creamy and tangy element. Finally, drizzle the bowl with olive oil and lemon juice for a light and refreshing meal that is both satisfying and healthy.

Mexican-Inspired Rice Bowl

For a grain bowl with a bit of a kick, try a Mexican-Inspired Rice Bowl. Start with a base of brown rice, which is rich in fiber and provides a hearty foundation for the bowl. Add black beans for a protein boost and corn for sweetness and texture. Diced avocado adds creaminess and healthy fats, while cherry tomatoes bring a burst of freshness. Grilled chicken serves as the primary protein source, offering a savory and filling component. To finish, top the bowl with a dollop of salsa, which adds a zesty and spicy flavor, and a squeeze of lime for a tangy finish. This bowl is not only delicious but also packed with nutrients, making it a perfect choice for a satisfying lunch.

Asian-Inspired Quinoa Bowl

For an Asian twist, try an Asian-Inspired Quinoa Bowl. Quinoa, known for its high protein content and nutty flavor, serves as the base for this bowl. Top the quinoa with edamame, which adds a pop of green color and a good source of protein. Shredded carrots contribute sweetness and crunch, while sliced bell peppers add vibrant color and a mild, sweet flavor. Grilled tofu serves as the main protein, offering a slightly chewy texture and a neutral flavor that absorbs the dressing well. Dress the bowl with a sesame ginger dressing for an Asian flair that ties all the ingredients together. The combination of flavors and textures in this bowl makes it a delightful and healthy lunch option.

Sandwiches And Wraps

Sandwiches and wraps are classic lunch items that can be easily adapted for an OMAD (One Meal A Day) lifestyle. They are not only portable and easy to prepare but also offer a versatile canvas for a variety of ingredients, ensuring your meals remain interesting and satisfying.

Turkey and Avocado Club Sandwich: This sandwich is a hearty and flavorful option that combines the best of savory and creamy textures. Start with whole-grain bread, which provides a wholesome and fiber-rich base. Layer on slices of turkey breast, known for its lean protein and low-fat content. Add creamy avocado slices, rich in healthy fats and vitamins, which not only enhance the nutritional value but also contribute a delightful creaminess. Top with crispy bacon strips for a savory crunch, fresh lettuce for a crisp bite, and juicy tomato slices for a burst of freshness. To finish, spread a little mayonnaise or mustard on the bread for added moisture and flavor. This turkey and avocado club sandwich is both filling and nutritious, making it an excellent choice for an OMAD meal.

Falafel Wrap: For a vegetarian option that's equally satisfying, consider a falafel wrap. Use whole-wheat tortillas, which offer a healthier alternative to white flour tortillas, providing more fiber and nutrients. Fill the wrap with crispy falafel balls, made from ground chickpeas and spices, which are a great source of plant-based protein and fiber. Add hummus for a creamy texture and additional protein. Shredded lettuce, tomatoes, and cucumbers bring in freshness and crunch. To elevate the flavor, drizzle with tzatziki sauce, a yogurt-based sauce with cucumber, garlic, and herbs, adding a tangy and refreshing zest to the wrap. This falafel wrap is not only delicious but also packed with nutrients, making it a perfect option for a balanced OMAD meal.

Grilled Veggie and Hummus Panini: For a warm and comforting option, a grilled veggie and hummus panini is a fantastic choice. Start by grilling a selection of your favorite vegetables such as zucchini, eggplant, and bell peppers. These vegetables become tender and develop a smoky flavor when grilled, making them incredibly tasty. Layer the grilled veggies with a generous spread of hummus on ciabatta bread. Hummus, made from blended chickpeas, provides a creamy and flavorful base that complements the vegetables perfectly. Press the sandwich in a panini maker until the bread is toasted and the veggies are warm. The result is a deliciously warm and hearty panini that's both nutritious and satisfying.

Soups and stews are more than just delicious meals; they offer warmth and nourishment, making them ideal choices for anyone looking to prepare meals in advance. These dishes can be made in large batches, allowing for easy portioning and reheating throughout the week, which is particularly beneficial for those practicing One Meal a Day (OMAD). By incorporating a diverse range of ingredients, soups and stews ensure a balanced meal packed with nutrients.

One classic example is the Hearty Beef Stew. This dish features tender chunks of beef, potatoes, carrots, and peas, all simmered together in a rich, savory broth. The slow cooking process allows the flavors to meld beautifully, resulting in a warm and satisfying meal that is especially comforting on colder days. The beef provides ample protein, while the vegetables contribute vitamins and minerals, making it a well-rounded option for your OMAD.

For a lighter alternative, consider the Chicken and Vegetable Soup. This recipe highlights lean chicken breast combined with a colorful medley of vegetables such as carrots, celery, and spinach, all simmered in a flavorful chicken broth. This soup is not only refreshing but also packed with nutrients, making it a great choice for those looking to enjoy a wholesome meal without feeling overly heavy. The broth is hydrating and can be easily customized with different herbs and spices, enhancing the overall flavor profile.

Another hearty option is the Lentil and Sausage Stew. This dish combines protein-rich lentils with spicy sausage, tomatoes, and nutritious kale, creating a filling and nutritious meal. The lentils add a significant amount of fiber, helping to keep you satisfied, while the sausage contributes depth of flavor and richness. This stew is perfect for meal prep, as it stores well and tastes even better the next day when the flavors have had time to develop.

CHAPTER FIVE

DINNER-INSPIRED OMAD RECIPES

One-Pot Meals

One-pot meals are an excellent option for those following the One Meal a Day (OMAD) lifestyle, offering a simple and efficient cooking experience. These dishes require minimal cleanup, making them ideal for busy schedules while still providing the satisfying and diverse flavors that are essential for a single daily meal.

The beauty of one-pot meals lies in their versatility. They allow you to combine a variety of ingredients, which not only enhances the flavors but also ensures a well-rounded meal. When cooked together, the ingredients share their tastes, resulting in a harmonious blend that delights the palate. Whether you opt for hearty stews, savory casseroles, or quick skillet dinners, there's a one-pot recipe for every preference.

For instance, consider a chicken and vegetable stir-fry, which can be whipped up in mere minutes using just one pan. Start with your choice of protein—chicken, tofu, or even shrimp—and add a colorful array of seasonal vegetables. Bell peppers, broccoli, and snap peas not only provide vibrant color but also contribute important nutrients. Toss everything in a flavorful sauce—like teriyaki, garlic soy, or a spicy chili mix—and stir-fry until cooked through. This approach yields a nutritious, satisfying meal packed with protein and fiber.

One-pot meals also shine when it comes to customization. You can easily adapt recipes based on what you have available in your pantry or fridge. For instance, if you have leftover grains, beans, or lentils, they can be tossed into the mix for added texture and nutrition. This flexibility not only helps in reducing food waste but also encourages creativity in the kitchen, allowing you to experiment with different spices and flavors.

Additionally, one-pot meals are particularly beneficial for meal prep. Preparing a large batch at the beginning of the week can save time and energy on busy days. Simply reheat your meal when it's time to eat, ensuring you have a nutritious option ready to go. This method not only simplifies your daily routine but also helps you stick to your OMAD plan by eliminating the temptation to snack throughout the day.

Roasted And Baked Dishes

Roasting and baking are two exceptional cooking methods that elevate the natural flavors of ingredients, making them ideal for your One Meal a Day (OMAD) dinner. These techniques not only provide a hearty and satisfying meal but also allow you to create dishes that feel indulgent while remaining nutritious.

One of the standout features of roasting is its ability to caramelize the sugars in vegetables, enhancing their sweetness and adding depth to the overall flavor. For instance, consider a roasted chicken paired with an array of root vegetables like carrots, potatoes, and parsnips. This dish is straightforward to prepare; simply season the chicken with your choice of herbs—such as rosemary or thyme—add a drizzle of olive oil, and arrange the chopped vegetables around the bird. Once in the oven, the heat transforms these simple ingredients into a rich, aromatic meal. The chicken becomes tender and juicy, while the vegetables absorb the savory juices, resulting in a delicious medley of flavors. Best of all, this meal can be enjoyed warm straight from the oven, or you can savor the leftovers the next day, adding convenience to your dining experience.

Baked dishes also offer incredible versatility for OMAD dinners. Casseroles, like lasagna or stuffed peppers, can be prepared in advance, allowing you to save time and effort. These dishes often combine layers of wholesome ingredients, making them both filling and nutritious. A classic lasagna, for example, can be packed with vegetables, lean proteins, and whole-grain noodles, then layered with a flavorful tomato sauce and a blend of cheeses. After baking, you have a comforting dish that is perfect for a hearty meal.

Stuffed peppers, on the other hand, are another delightful baked option. They can be filled with a mixture of quinoa, black beans, and diced tomatoes, then topped with spices and cheese before being baked to perfection. The peppers become tender while retaining their structure, making each bite a burst of flavor.

Pasta And Noodle Dishes

Pasta and noodle dishes are incredibly versatile, making them a popular choice for dinner across many cultures. Their adaptability allows for a wide range of ingredients, flavors, and cooking methods, catering to various dietary preferences and needs. Whether you prefer whole grain options or gluten-free varieties, pasta can be modified to fit into different meal plans, including those focused on health and nutrition.

For individuals following an OMAD (One Meal a Day) lifestyle, one-pot pasta recipes stand out as a particularly appealing option. These dishes combine the cooking of the pasta and sauce in a single pot, which not only saves time but also minimizes cleanup. The simplicity of this method allows for quick preparation without compromising on taste or nutrition. For example, a classic spaghetti dish can be elevated by incorporating fresh vegetables, such as spinach, bell peppers, or zucchini, along with lean proteins like grilled chicken, shrimp, or tofu. A homemade sauce made from ripe tomatoes, garlic, and herbs can add a nutritious punch, making the meal both satisfying and wholesome.

Asian-inspired noodle dishes also fit seamlessly within the OMAD framework. Quick to prepare, these meals often feature stir-fried soba noodles or rice noodles, which can be tossed with an array of vegetables and protein sources. Adding elements like garlic, ginger, and sesame oil enhances the flavor, while vegetables such as bok choy, carrots, and snap peas add texture and nutrients. The incorporation of sauces, such as soy sauce or hoisin, can provide depth and umami, ensuring that your meal is not only healthy but also packed with flavor.

Both pasta and noodle dishes can be tailored to suit individual tastes, making them an excellent choice for meal prep. You can easily batch-cook a variety of sauces or stir-fried ingredients to have on hand, allowing for effortless assembly during your designated meal time. Furthermore, these dishes lend themselves well to experimentation; incorporating seasonal produce or different spices can refresh the meal and keep it exciting week after week.

Grilling and BBQ cooking extend far beyond the summer months; they can transform your One Meal a Day (OMAD) experience into a delightful culinary adventure at any time of the year. The unique smoky flavor imparted by grilling enhances the taste of meats, vegetables, and even fruits, making every bite memorable.

One of the great joys of grilling is its versatility. Whether you're firing up the grill for juicy chicken thighs, succulent ribs, or vibrant vegetable skewers, there's something satisfying about the entire process. Grilled meats not only offer rich flavors but can also be healthier than other cooking methods. As the food cooks, excess fats drip away, leaving behind a leaner, more nutritious meal.

To maximize flavor, consider marinating your proteins ahead of time. A simple marinade can transform ordinary cuts of meat into extraordinary dishes. Ingredients such as olive oil, garlic, fresh herbs, and spices can create a depth of flavor that is both exciting and satisfying. Marinate your proteins for at least an hour—or overnight for even more intense flavor—before grilling. This allows the marinade to penetrate the meat, making it tender and infused with delicious seasonings.

Vegetables are also a fantastic addition to your grill. The high heat caramelizes their natural sugars, resulting in an appealing texture and enhanced flavor. Think bell peppers, zucchini, asparagus, and mushrooms; they're all excellent choices. Toss them with a little olive oil and your favorite spices, and let the grill work its magic. Adding grilled fruits, like peaches or pineapples, can introduce a sweet contrast to your savory dishes, creating a well-rounded meal that excites the palate.

Pair your grilled items with fresh salads or whole grain sides to complement the flavors and boost the nutritional value of your OMAD dinner. A vibrant salad with mixed greens, cherry tomatoes, and a tangy vinaigrette can provide a refreshing counterpoint to the smoky richness of grilled meats. Whole grains like quinoa or farro can add substance and a satisfying chewiness to your meal.

CHAPTER SIX

SNACKS AND SIDES FOR OMAD

Healthy Snack Options

Snacking can play a vital role in maintaining your energy levels and curbing cravings, especially when following the One Meal a Day (OMAD) diet. While the OMAD approach focuses on consuming all your daily calories in a single meal, having nutrient-dense snacks can be beneficial for those moments when hunger strikes. Here are some healthy snack options that can help you stay satisfied while adhering to your dietary goals.

Nuts and Seeds

A handful of nuts or seeds can serve as a powerhouse of nutrients. Almonds, walnuts, chia seeds, and flaxseeds are excellent choices, as they are rich in healthy fats, protein, and fiber. These nutrients not only help curb hunger but also provide sustained energy throughout your day. Just a small serving can go a long way in keeping your cravings at bay, making them an ideal snack option for OMAD practitioners.

Greek Yogurt

Greek yogurt stands out as a protein-rich snack that also contains probiotics, which are beneficial for gut health. You can enjoy it plain for a low-sugar option, or add fresh berries for natural sweetness and antioxidants. This combination not only satisfies your taste buds but also offers a good balance of protein and carbohydrates, perfect for keeping energy levels steady.

Vegetable Sticks with Hummus

Pairing crunchy vegetable sticks with hummus creates a satisfying and nutritious snack. Carrot, celery, and cucumber sticks are low in calories and high in fiber, making them excellent choices for snacking. When dipped in hummus, they gain a boost of protein and healthy fats, creating a delicious and filling option that can help you avoid high-calorie processed snacks.

Hard-Boiled Eggs

For a quick and portable source of protein, hard-boiled eggs are hard to beat. They can be seasoned with various herbs or spices for added flavor, and their convenience makes them an ideal snack option when you're on the go. Eggs are not only nutritious but also versatile, as they can be paired with other foods or enjoyed on their own.

Cheese Cubes

Cheese can be a great addition to your snacking routine due to its high calcium and protein content. Choosing small portions of cheese can help you manage your calorie intake while still enjoying the rich flavors. Whether you opt for cheddar, mozzarella, or another favorite, cheese can provide a satisfying treat that complements other healthy snacks.

Vegetable Side Dishes

Incorporating vegetable side dishes into your main meal is essential for ensuring a balanced diet rich in vitamins, minerals, and fiber. Vegetables not only enhance the nutritional profile of your meals but also add vibrant colors and flavors, making your plate more appealing. Here are some delicious options to consider:

Roasted Vegetables: Roasting is one of the best methods to bring out the natural sweetness of vegetables. When you roast vegetables, the high heat caramelizes their sugars, resulting in a rich, complex flavor. A delightful combination to try is bell peppers, zucchini, broccoli, and carrots. Simply chop them into bite-sized pieces, toss them in olive oil, and season with your favorite herbs such as rosemary, thyme, or oregano. Spread the mixture on a baking sheet and roast in the oven until tender and slightly browned. The result is a flavorful side dish that complements a variety of main courses.

Steamed Greens: Leafy greens like spinach, kale, or Swiss chard are nutritional powerhouses, packed with vitamins A, C, and K, along with important minerals like iron and calcium. Steaming is an excellent cooking method for greens as it helps retain their vibrant color and nutritional value. To prepare, simply steam the greens until they are wilted yet bright, about 3-5 minutes. For added flavor, toss them with a splash of lemon juice and a pinch of salt or your favorite seasoning. This simple dish not only provides a burst of color but also boosts your meal's nutrient content.

Cauliflower Rice: If you're looking for a low-carb alternative to traditional rice, cauliflower rice is an excellent choice. It's versatile and can easily take on the flavors of the spices or other ingredients you mix in. To make cauliflower rice, pulse raw cauliflower florets in a food processor until they resemble grains. Sauté the cauliflower rice in a pan with olive oil, garlic, and any additional vegetables or spices you like. This healthy alternative pairs well with stir-fries or can be used as a base for various dishes.

Grilled Asparagus: Asparagus is not only delicious but also rich in vitamins A, C, and K. Grilling enhances its natural flavors while giving it a delightful char. To prepare grilled asparagus, simply trim the tough ends, toss them with olive oil, salt, and pepper, and place them on a preheated grill. Cook until tender and slightly charred, usually about 5-7 minutes. This simple preparation method highlights the asparagus's unique taste and adds a touch of sophistication to your meal.

Protein-Rich Sides

When following an OMAD (One Meal a Day) diet, ensuring that your meal is nutrient-dense is essential, especially when it comes to protein. Protein plays a crucial role in muscle maintenance, satiety, and overall health. Incorporating protein-rich side dishes can enhance your meal experience while providing the necessary nutrients. Here are some delicious and nutritious options to consider:

Quinoa stands out as a powerhouse grain. Unlike many other grains, quinoa is a complete protein, meaning it contains all nine essential amino acids required by the body. This makes it an excellent choice for anyone looking to increase their protein intake. Additionally, quinoa is gluten-free, making it suitable for those with gluten sensitivities. Its nutty flavor and fluffy texture allow it to be a versatile addition to your meal. You can cook quinoa in vegetable or chicken broth for added flavor, or mix it with herbs like parsley, cilantro, or mint. It can also serve as a base for salads, providing both protein and a satisfying texture.

Chickpeas are another fantastic option for protein-rich sides. These legumes are not only high in protein but also packed with fiber, making them a filling choice. One of the most enjoyable ways to prepare chickpeas is by roasting them. Roasting gives them a crunchy texture and a satisfying snack-like quality. Simply toss canned or cooked chickpeas with olive oil, salt, and your favorite spices before roasting until crispy. Roasted chickpeas can be enjoyed on their own or sprinkled over salads and grain bowls for an added crunch. Their versatility also allows for creative flavoring—try adding garlic powder, paprika, or even cayenne for a kick.

Grilled Chicken or Fish provides another excellent source of lean protein. Chicken breast and fish fillets, such as salmon or tilapia, are both low in fat and high in protein, making them ideal for a healthy diet. Grilling not only enhances the flavor but also keeps the cooking method healthy by allowing excess fat to drip away. You can season these proteins with a variety of marinades or dry rubs—think lemon and herbs for chicken or a spicy marinade for fish—to suit your palate. These grilled options can be served alongside your main dish or added to salads, providing both flavor and a satisfying protein boost.

Low-Carb Options

For those embracing a low-carb approach within the One Meal a Day (OMAD) framework, selecting side dishes that are lower in carbohydrates is essential for maintaining stable energy levels and supporting effective weight management. Here are some delicious low-carb ideas that can complement your main dish while keeping carb counts low.

Zucchini Noodles (Zoodles): One of the most popular low-carb alternatives to traditional pasta is zucchini noodles, often referred to as zoodles. These are made by spiralizing fresh zucchini into thin strands that resemble spaghetti. Zoodles are incredibly versatile; they can be sautéed lightly with olive oil, garlic, and your choice of herbs for added flavor. Alternatively, they can be served raw in salads, absorbing dressings beautifully. Their mild flavor makes them an excellent base for sauces, from marinara to creamy Alfredo, allowing you to enjoy a satisfying pasta-like dish without the carbs.

Stuffed Bell Peppers: Another fantastic low-carb option is stuffed bell peppers. By hollowing out vibrant bell peppers and filling them with a hearty mixture of ground meat (such as turkey, beef, or chicken), vegetables, and a blend of spices, you can create a colorful and nutritious dish. The sweetness of the bell peppers pairs wonderfully with the savory filling, making for a comforting meal that is both satisfying and low in carbohydrates. You can also customize the stuffing with ingredients like cauliflower rice or quinoa for added texture without significantly increasing carb content.

Eggplant Parmesan: Traditional eggplant Parmesan is often breaded and fried, but you can make a low-carb version that retains all the delicious flavors while eliminating the excess carbs. Start by slicing eggplant and baking it until tender. Layer the baked eggplant with marinara sauce and plenty of cheese—such as mozzarella or Parmesan—for a rich and cheesy dish. This approach provides the satisfaction of a classic Italian favorite without the carbs associated with breading.

You can even add fresh basil or oregano to enhance the flavor profile.

CHAPTER SEVEN

DESSERTS AND TREATS FOR OMAD

Guilt-Free Desserts

Guilt-free desserts are the perfect solution for satisfying your sweet tooth while maintaining a healthier lifestyle. These treats are crafted with wholesome ingredients that nourish your body, allowing you to indulge without the usual pangs of regret. By substituting traditional refined sugars with natural sweeteners, such as honey or maple syrup, guilt-free desserts provide a delicious way to enjoy sweets without compromising your health goals.

One standout option is chocolate avocado mousse, which combines the creamy richness of ripe avocados with cocoa powder for a decadent flavor. Avocados are packed with healthy fats, vitamins, and fiber, making them an excellent base for this indulgent dessert. Simply blend ripe avocados with unsweetened cocoa powder and a touch of your preferred natural sweetener. The result is a rich, silky mousse that satisfies chocolate cravings while offering nutritional benefits. Not only is this dessert delicious, but it also supports heart health and helps maintain steady energy levels.

Another favorite among guilt-free dessert enthusiasts is chia seed pudding. Chia seeds are tiny powerhouses of nutrition, rich in omega-3 fatty acids, fiber, and antioxidants. To prepare chia seed pudding, mix chia seeds with almond milk (or any milk of your choice) and let the mixture soak overnight in the refrigerator. This allows the seeds to absorb the liquid and swell, creating a delightful pudding-like consistency. For added sweetness, you can incorporate natural ingredients like ripe bananas, fresh berries, or a drizzle of honey. Top it off with your choice of nuts or seeds for a delightful crunch and additional nutrients.

These guilt-free desserts not only cater to health-conscious individuals but also appeal to anyone looking to enjoy sweets without the burden of excessive calories or artificial ingredients. By embracing natural alternatives and whole food ingredients, you can create a variety of desserts that feel indulgent yet are nourishing.

Fruit-Based Treats

Fruit-based treats are an excellent way to indulge your sweet tooth while reaping the health benefits that fruits offer. Rich in vitamins, minerals, and antioxidants, fruits can enhance your overall well-being. They can be enjoyed fresh or transformed into delightful desserts that satisfy cravings without compromising health.

One simple yet refreshing option is a seasonal fruit salad. Combine a variety of fresh fruits like strawberries, blueberries, kiwi, and melons for a colorful, nutritious dish. This salad is not only visually appealing but also packed with essential nutrients and natural sweetness. You can elevate the flavor by adding a squeeze of lime juice or a sprinkle of mint, making it a perfect side dish or a light dessert.

If you're looking for a creamy treat, consider making banana ice cream. This dessert is incredibly easy to prepare and serves as a fantastic alternative to traditional ice cream. To make it, freeze ripe bananas, then blend them until smooth. The result is a creamy, soft-serve-like texture without any added sugars or dairy. You can customize this treat by adding cocoa powder for a chocolate flavor, or peanut butter for a nutty richness. Feel free to mix in other frozen fruits like strawberries or mangoes for a fruity twist. This banana ice cream is not only delicious but also a healthier option that fits seamlessly into your dietary choices.

Another comforting option is baked fruit. Baked apples or pears make for a warm and satisfying dessert, especially on cooler days. To prepare, simply core the fruit and sprinkle it with cinnamon and a drizzle of honey. Bake until the fruit is tender and fragrant. The natural sweetness of the fruit, combined with the warmth of cinnamon, creates a comforting dessert that feels indulgent while still being wholesome. This baked fruit can be served on its own or alongside a dollop of yogurt for added creaminess.

Protein-Packed Desserts

Incorporating protein into your desserts is a great way to enhance their nutritional value while satisfying your sweet tooth. Protein-packed desserts not only help keep you feeling fuller for longer but also support muscle recovery and overall health. Ingredients like Greek yogurt, protein powder, and nuts are excellent choices for boosting the protein content of your favorite treats.

One delightful option is Greek yogurt parfaits. These parfaits are layered with creamy Greek yogurt, crunchy granola, and fresh berries, creating a delicious and nutritious dessert. The yogurt provides a rich source of protein and probiotics, promoting gut health, while the granola adds texture and fiber. Berries, on the other hand, contribute antioxidants and vitamins, making this dessert not just filling but also wholesome.

For chocolate lovers, protein brownies made with black beans or chickpeas are an innovative twist on the classic treat. While it may sound unusual to use beans in a dessert, when blended with cocoa powder and a natural sweetener, they transform into fudgy brownies that are surprisingly high in protein and fiber. The beans lend a moist texture, while the cocoa provides that rich chocolate flavor you crave. These brownies can satisfy your chocolate cravings while aligning with your health goals, making them an excellent option for an indulgent yet nutritious dessert.

Another easy and convenient protein-packed dessert is energy balls. These no-bake treats are incredibly simple to prepare and can be customized to your taste preferences. Typically made with oats, nut butter, protein powder, and a touch of honey, energy balls offer a well-rounded snack that is portable and satisfying. The combination of carbohydrates from the oats, healthy fats from the nut butter, and protein from the protein powder provides a balanced energy boost, making them ideal for those following an OMAD (One Meal a Day) routine.

In addition to being nutritious, these protein-packed desserts can be tailored to suit various dietary preferences, such as gluten-free or vegan options. With a little creativity and the right ingredients, you can enjoy delicious desserts that not only satisfy your sweet tooth but also contribute positively to your health and well-being.

Indulgent But Healthy Treats

Indulgent yet healthy treats allow you to satisfy your cravings for something rich without compromising your commitment to nutrition. These delightful options can be both satisfying and guilt-free, making them perfect for any occasion.

One of the best examples of a healthy indulgence is dark chocolate. Unlike its milk chocolate counterpart, dark chocolate is typically lower in sugar and packed with antioxidants, which can help combat free radicals in the body. The higher the cocoa content, the more beneficial compounds you get. A few squares of high-quality dark chocolate can serve as a perfect after-dinner treat, offering a rich flavor that feels indulgent while being kinder to your health. For a fancier twist, consider making dark chocolate-covered strawberries. Simply melt dark chocolate and dip fresh strawberries in it, then let them cool until the chocolate hardens. This not only makes for an elegant dessert but also combines the sweetness of fruit with the richness of chocolate, resulting in a treat that feels luxurious yet is full of nutrients.

Another excellent option for a healthy indulgent treat is a no-bake cheesecake made from cashews. By blending soaked cashews with coconut cream, lemon juice, and a touch of your favorite natural sweetener, you can create a creamy filling that mimics traditional cheesecake but is entirely plant-based. The result is a decadent dessert that is rich and satisfying, perfect for those who crave something sweet. This cheesecake can be poured into a crust made from crushed nuts and dates for an added layer of flavor and texture. It's an easy recipe that requires minimal effort but yields impressive results.

For an even simpler treat, consider making yogurt parfaits. Layer Greek yogurt with your favorite fruits, nuts, and a drizzle of honey or maple syrup for a delightful snack that feels indulgent. The creaminess of the yogurt combined with the sweetness of the fruits and the crunch of the nuts creates a satisfying treat that nourishes your body.

THE END